Breathe Deep

"A Guide to Residency in Pulmonary Medicine and Beyond"

Dr Ravi Kumar Sharma
MBBS(CNMC Kolkata)
PGDFM(CMC Vellore)
DTCD(PGIMS Rohtak)
DNB(NITRD New Delhi)
Assistant Professor
Dept. Of Respiratory Medicine
GMC Haldwani, UK India

"The tallest oak in the forest was once just a little nut that held its ground."

Although the path may be challenging and filled with moments of doubt and exhaustion, perseverance, determination, and resilience will lead to growth and eventual success. Every step, even the small or difficult ones, contributes to the strength and wisdom you will gain as you evolve into a skilled and compassionate physician.

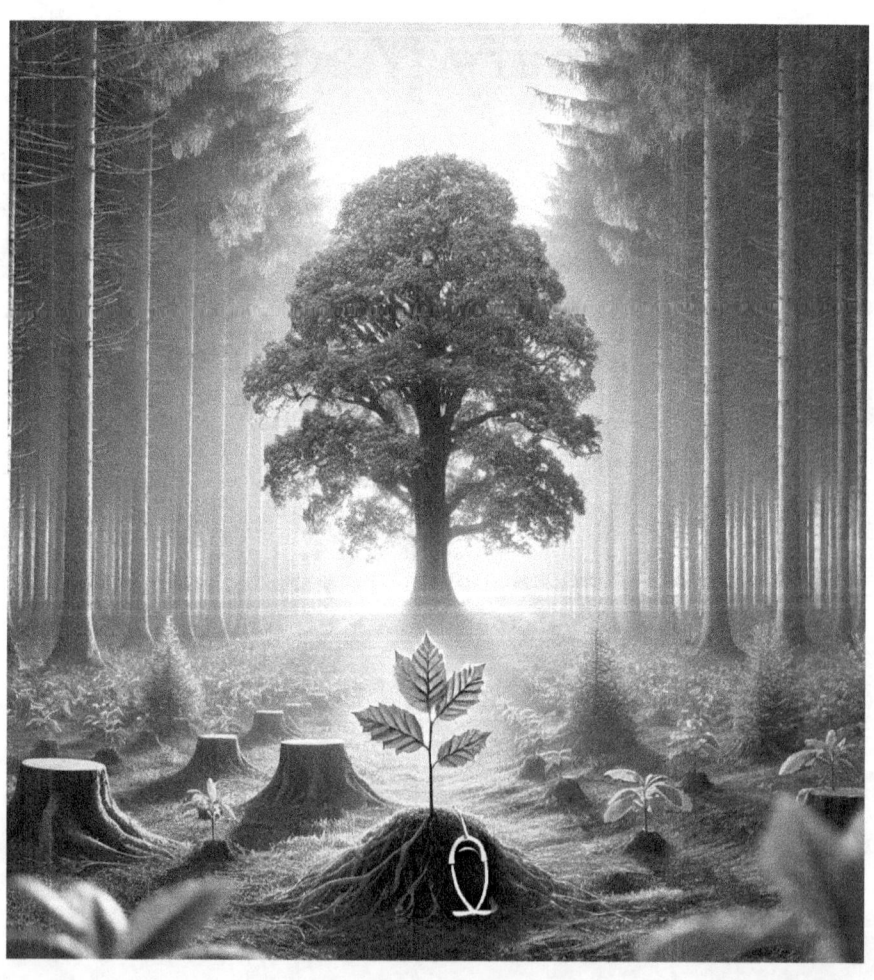

Breathe Deep

"A Guide to Residency in Pulmonary Medicine and Beyond"

*Dedicated to Shree Shyam Ji,
My Parents, Siblings,
My Wife Dr Ravita and
My Son Srijan Sharma (Sam)*

Contents

Chapter 1 : Role of Pulmonologist and TB Physician in Current Indian and Worldwide Perspective

Chapter 2; Career and Financial Aspects of Pulmonologists and TB Physicians: Role and Income Perspective in the Current Indian and Worldwide Context

Chapter 3. Subject specific objectives

Chapter 4.Syllabus as per NMC (India) Curriculum

Chapter 5. Teaching and learning methods

Chapter 6; Recommended Books Our eyes cannot see what Brain doesn't KNOW

Chapter 7; Standard Pulmonary Disease definitions

Chapter 8; How to Learn in MD Pulmonary Medicine Residency Despite a Hectic Work Schedule

Chapter 9; Ethical and Humanitarian Implications of Poor Training in MD Pulmonary Medicine Residency in the Indian Context

Chapter 10; Legal Implications of Poor Training in MD Pulmonary Medicine Residency in the Indian Context

Chapter 11; How to Enjoy an MD Residency Program Despite Hectic Work Hours

Chapter 12; Importance of Basic Statistical Knowledge in MD Residency Programs

Chapter 13: A Code of Ethics and Professional Conduct for Resident Doctors

Chapter 14; Message for MD Residents and Concluding Remarks

Preface;

The purpose of PG education is to create specialists who would provide high quality health care and advance the cause of science through research & training. Evolution of critical care medicine makes it imperative that the post graduates are trained in the basic principles of Pulmonary Medicine as applied to critical care. The person shall be abreast with the recent advances and developments in the specialty of Pulmonary Medicine. It is expected that the person will develop a spirit of enquiry and get oriented to apply recent advances and medical evidence to the practice of pulmonary medicine. He would also grasp the fundamentals of research methodology. Medical Science is dynamic with a continuous enhancement of knowledge. The process of acquiring knowledge and skills continues even after formal education. The syllabus to be covered during post graduate training in Pulmonary Medicine given below is designed to develop a sound and scientific foundation. It is intended to serve as a guide to impart basic knowledge and develop skills and does not impose any limits to expansion beyond the areas listed. The purpose of this book is to provide young budding Resident Doctors in Pulmonary medicine to achieve defined outcomes through learning and assessment. This book is going to work as a guide to help them understand the beautiful journey of residency period with importance of day to day challenges. Hope you enjoy this booklet and my best wishes to all new resident physicians. Please share you feedback and suggestions for further improvement.Wishing again all of the new budding Resident a happy and amazing Journey in Medical Learning.

Dr Ravi Kumar Sharma
Date; 20.12.2024
Place; Haldwani , Uttarakhand India
Email; drravi133@gmail.com

CHAPTER 1 : ROLE OF PULMONOLOGIST AND TB PHYSICIAN IN CURRENT INDIAN AND WORLDWIDE PERSPECTIVE

1. Introduction

The roles of pulmonologists and tuberculosis (TB) physicians are crucial in managing respiratory diseases, with a particular emphasis on tuberculosis, which remains a significant global health challenge. As specialists in respiratory medicine, these doctors are involved in diagnosing, treating, and managing a wide range of pulmonary conditions, including TB. Their roles are vital in both the Indian and global healthcare systems, especially in regions with high disease burden.

2. Pulmonologist's Role in the Healthcare System

Pulmonologists are medical professionals who specialize in the diagnosis and treatment of diseases related to the lungs and respiratory system. Their role has expanded significantly, particularly in managing chronic respiratory diseases, infections, and critical care.

2.1 Areas of Expertise

- Chronic Obstructive Pulmonary Disease (COPD): Pulmonologists are experts in managing COPD, a leading cause of morbidity and mortality worldwide, which requires long-term management strategies.
- Asthma and Allergic Disorders: Diagnosing and managing asthma, bronchial allergies, and other pulmonary disorders.
- Lung Cancer: Early detection and management of lung cancer, including the latest advancements in oncology and targeted therapies.
- Pulmonary Infections: Diagnosing and treating acute infections like pneumonia, COVID-19, and TB.

- Critical Care: Pulmonologists play a key role in managing patients with severe respiratory distress, including mechanical ventilation and ECMO in intensive care units.

2.2 Key Responsibilities

- Diagnosis and Treatment: The pulmonologist is responsible for diagnosing lung diseases through various tests, including chest X-rays, CT scans, pulmonary function tests, and bronchoscopy. Treatment may involve medications, therapies, or procedures such as intubation or lung surgery.
- Prevention and Health Promotion: Educating the public about smoking cessation, pollution control, and respiratory hygiene, which are critical in the prevention of respiratory diseases.

3. Role of TB Physicians in India and Worldwide

Tuberculosis is one of the oldest known infectious diseases, and despite advances in medicine, it remains a major health threat, particularly in low- and middle-income countries. TB physicians specialize in the diagnosis, treatment, and management of TB and its complications.

3.1 Global TB Burden and India's Situation

- Global Perspective: According to the World Health Organization (WHO), TB is one of the top 10 causes of death globally. In 2022, an estimated 10.6 million people fell ill with TB, with the highest burden in India, China, and Indonesia.
- Indian Context: India is the country with the highest TB burden, accounting for a quarter of global cases. Factors contributing to this include overcrowded living conditions, malnutrition, and the HIV epidemic. India's National TB Elimination Program (NTEP) aims to eliminate TB by 2025, which presents an enormous challenge.

3.2 Key Responsibilities of TB Physicians

- Diagnosis: TB physicians are responsible for diagnosing TB through microbiological tests (e.g., sputum smear microscopy, GeneXpert) and imaging techniques. In India, they often deal with drug-resistant TB (DR-TB), which requires specialized diagnostic tools and prolonged treatment.
- Treatment and Management: Managing both drug-sensitive and drug-resistant TB is a primary responsibility. This involves initiating the correct anti-TB regimen, closely monitoring treatment adherence, and managing side effects.
- Public Health and Community Engagement: TB physicians also play a role in public health initiatives, providing education on TB prevention, improving awareness, and combating stigma. They work with health systems to ensure TB patients complete their treatment, preventing further spread.
- Collaboration in TB Research: TB physicians often collaborate in research to develop new diagnostics, drugs, and vaccines to address the global TB crisis, especially with the increasing burden of drug-resistant TB.

3.3 Challenges in TB Care

- Drug-Resistant Tuberculosis (DR-TB): The rising incidence of multi-drug-resistant TB (MDR-TB) and extensively drug-resistant TB (XDR-TB) poses significant challenges. These conditions require prolonged and more complex treatment regimens, with a higher risk of treatment failure.
- TB-HIV Co-infection: TB is the leading cause of death among people living with HIV, complicating TB diagnosis and treatment.
- Access to Care: In many countries, especially in rural and underserved regions, access to timely and adequate TB diagnosis and treatment remains a challenge.

4. Collaborative Role of Pulmonologists and TB Physicians

Both pulmonologists and TB physicians often work closely in treating patients with complex pulmonary diseases, including TB. In areas with high TB prevalence, pulmonologists are typically involved in the early diagnosis of TB, especially in cases with atypical presentations.

4.1 Joint Efforts in TB and Respiratory Disease Management

- Integrated Approaches: Both specialists often coordinate care, particularly in cases of TB-related lung damage or when managing co-morbidities like COPD and TB.
- Post-TB Care: Pulmonologists play a crucial role in post-TB management, addressing lung damage or respiratory complications following successful TB treatment.

5. Technological Advancements and Their Impact

The rise of digital health technologies has significantly impacted the role of both pulmonologists and TB physicians. Telemedicine, for example, has enhanced the ability of TB physicians in rural and remote areas to provide consultations and follow-up care.

5.1 Innovations in TB Treatment

- Shorter Regimens for Drug-Resistant TB: Newer drug regimens are making it easier to treat drug-resistant TB, with the World Health Organization recommending shorter and more effective treatments.
- New Diagnostic Tools: Advances in molecular diagnostic techniques, such as the GeneXpert, have improved the speed and accuracy of TB diagnosis, allowing for earlier detection and treatment.

SUMMARY

Pulmonologists and TB physicians are at the forefront of managing respiratory diseases, especially tuberculosis. In both India and worldwide, their role is critical in combating TB, particularly in the face of rising drug resistance and co-infection with HIV. Collaboration, continued research, and adoption of new technologies are key to tackling the growing burden of respiratory diseases and TB, with the ultimate goal of improving patient outcomes and achieving TB elimination.

CHAPTER 2; CAREER AND FINANCIAL ASPECTS OF PULMONOLOGISTS AND TB PHYSICIANS: ROLE AND INCOME PERSPECTIVE IN THE CURRENT INDIAN AND WORLDWIDE CONTEXT

1. Role of Pulmonologists and TB Physicians:

Pulmonologists and TB (Tuberculosis) physicians play a critical role in the healthcare system, focusing on the diagnosis, treatment, and management of respiratory diseases, including chronic conditions like Chronic Obstructive Pulmonary Disease (COPD), asthma, and lung infections, as well as infectious diseases such as tuberculosis (TB). Their roles have evolved significantly in both the Indian and global contexts, given the rising burden of respiratory diseases and emerging health challenges.

Pulmonologists:

- Diagnosis and Management: Pulmonologists diagnose and manage a wide range of respiratory disorders, including asthma, COPD, interstitial lung diseases, lung cancer, and sleep apnea. They use a variety of diagnostic tools such as chest X-rays, CT scans, pulmonary function tests (PFTs), and bronchoscopy.
- Critical Care: Pulmonologists often work in intensive care units (ICUs) to manage critically ill patients with respiratory failure, particularly those on ventilators or with severe cases of pneumonia or ARDS (acute respiratory distress syndrome).
- Prevention and Rehabilitation: They play an active role in public health by advising on smoking cessation, pollution control, and promoting lung health. Pulmonary rehabilitation programs for patients with chronic respiratory diseases are a significant part of their practice.

TB Physicians:

- Diagnosis and Treatment of TB: TB physicians specialize in the diagnosis and management of tuberculosis, which remains a global health challenge, especially in developing countries like India. They administer multi-drug regimens, manage drug-resistant TB (XDR-TB and MDR-TB), and address the complications associated with the disease.
- Public Health Initiatives: TB physicians are actively involved in TB control programs and campaigns, contributing to national and global efforts to eradicate the disease. In India, the Revised National Tuberculosis Control Program (RNTCP) is a major initiative where TB specialists have a significant role in implementing strategies.
- Research and Education: They contribute to TB research, especially in drug development, treatment protocols, and disease prevention strategies. They are also involved in educating communities and healthcare workers about TB transmission, symptoms, and preventive measures.

2. Career Path and Professional Development:

- Education and Training: To become a pulmonologist or TB physician, a medical degree (MBBS) is required, followed by postgraduate specialization. Pulmonologists typically pursue a Master of Medicine (MD) or a Diploma in Tuberculosis and Chest Diseases (DTCD), followed by a fellowship or further training in advanced respiratory care. TB physicians often focus on pulmonary medicine with specialized training in infectious diseases and TB management.
- Global Perspective: Pulmonologists and TB physicians have career opportunities worldwide, particularly in regions facing significant respiratory disease burdens. Developed countries, including the U.S., the UK, and Australia, offer advanced training, research, and clinical opportunities. In the developing world, such as India, pulmonologists and TB

specialists are in high demand to address the growing prevalence of both communicable and non-communicable lung diseases.
- Research and Teaching Opportunities: Both pulmonologists and TB specialists can pursue academic careers by engaging in research, teaching, and contributing to global health policies. International organizations, including the World Health Organization (WHO), frequently collaborate with these professionals on large-scale TB elimination projects and respiratory disease management programs.

3. Income Perspective:

The income of pulmonologists and TB physicians can vary significantly depending on factors such as geographical location, level of experience, type of practice (private vs. public), and professional reputation.

Income in India:

- Private Sector: Pulmonologists working in private hospitals or owning their own practice typically have higher earning potential. Fees for consultations, diagnostic procedures (such as PFTs, bronchoscopy), and specialized treatments can bring in substantial income. The average income of a pulmonologist in India can range from INR 12 lakhs to INR 30 lakhs annually, depending on their experience and reputation. Top-tier pulmonologists with significant patient loads and specialized expertise may earn upwards of INR 50 lakhs per year.
- Government Sector: Pulmonologists employed in government hospitals or public health sectors generally earn a fixed salary, which may range from INR 8 lakhs to INR 20 lakhs per year, depending on experience and rank. However, many government-employed pulmonologists supplement their income with private practice or consultations.

- TB Specialists: TB specialists, often employed in government-run TB control programs, may earn a salary ranging from INR 6 lakhs to INR 15 lakhs annually, depending on the position and level of responsibility. Income can be enhanced with private consultations and involvement in research or international health programs.

Income Worldwide:

- Developed Countries: Pulmonologists in the United States, the United Kingdom, and Australia generally earn much higher salaries due to the advanced healthcare systems and high demand for respiratory specialists. For example, a pulmonologist in the U.S. can earn anywhere between USD 200,000 to USD 400,000 annually, depending on experience, location, and type of practice.
- Income in the UK and Europe: In the UK, NHS-employed pulmonologists typically earn between GBP 60,000 to GBP 100,000 annually. Private practitioners or those with senior roles in major hospitals can earn more.
- Global Demand and Opportunities: With the rising global burden of diseases like COPD, asthma, and TB, there is increasing demand for pulmonologists and TB specialists in both developed and developing countries. This demand, combined with global health initiatives, creates opportunities for higher incomes, particularly in research, academia, and international organizations working on TB and respiratory health.

4. Challenges and Opportunities:

- Challenges in India: In India, pulmonologists and TB specialists face challenges such as inadequate infrastructure, limited access to advanced medical equipment, and gaps in awareness and healthcare resources. Additionally, the high burden of both communicable (TB) and non-communicable

diseases (COPD, asthma) places immense pressure on healthcare professionals.
- Opportunities for Growth: The growing burden of respiratory diseases in India and globally, coupled with advancements in treatment options and diagnostic technologies, presents ample career growth opportunities. Increased government focus on improving healthcare systems, particularly in respiratory care and TB eradication programs, offers stability and demand for specialists in this field.

SUMMARY:

Pulmonologists and TB physicians play an indispensable role in addressing respiratory health challenges, both in India and globally. While the income potential can vary depending on practice settings, experience, and geography, these professionals are integral to combating respiratory diseases. With increasing awareness, evolving treatment protocols, and research initiatives, the career outlook for pulmonologists and TB specialists is promising, offering both professional satisfaction and financial rewards.

CHAPTER 3. SUBJECT SPECIFIC OBJECTIVES

The primary goal of the MD course in Pulmonary Medicine is to produce post graduate clinicians able to provide health care in the field of pulmonary medicine.
It is expected that a physician qualified in Pulmonary Medicine at the end of the course should be
- Able to diagnose and treat pulmonary diseases,
- Take preventive and curative steps for these diseases in the community at all levels of health care.
- Qualify as a consultant and teacher in the subject.

Each student should obtain proficiency in the following domains during the period training:
1. Theoretical knowledge of different aspects of Pulmonary Medicine including the
status in health and disease.
2. Acquire clinical skills.
3. Acquire practical skills.
4. Management of emergencies including intensive care.
5. Preparation of thesis as per MCI/ NMC guidelines.
These involve patient management in the outpatient, inpatient and emergency situations, case presentations, didactic lectures, seminars, journal reviews, clinico-patholgical
conferences and mortality review meetings and working in the laboratories.

SUBJECT SPECIFIC COMPETENCIES
By the end of the course, the student should have acquired knowledge (cognitive domain), professionalism (affective domain) and skills (psychomotor domain) as given below:
A. Cognitive domain At the end of the MD course in Pulmonary Medicine, the students should be able to:
1. Demonstrate sound knowledge of common pulmonary diseases, their clinical Manifestations, including emergent situations and of investigative procedures To confirm their diagnosis. A

comprehensive knowledge of epidemiological Aspects of pulmonary diseases should be acquired.
2. Demonstrate comprehensive knowledge of various modes of therapy used in Treatment of pulmonary diseases.
3. Describe the mode of action of commonly used drugs, their doses, side-effects/ toxicity, indications and contra-indications and interactions.
4. Describe commonly used modes of management including medical and Surgical procedures available for treatment of various diseases and to offer a Comprehensive plan of management inclusive of national tuberculosis control Programme.
5. Manage common pulmonary emergencies and understand the basic of Intensive care in patients with pulmonary diseases.
6. Practice the field of pulmonary medicine ethically and assiduously, show Empathy and adopt a humane approach towards patients and their families.
7. Recognize the national priorities in pulmonary medicine and play an important Role in the implementation of national health programmes including Tuberculosis.
8. Demonstrate competence in medical management.
9. Should inculcate good reading habits and develop ability to search medical Literature and develop basic concept of medical research.

B. AFFECTIVE DOMAIN
1. Should be able to function as a part of a team, develop an attitude of cooperation with colleagues, and interact with the patient and the clinician or other colleagues to provide the best possible diagnosis or opinion.
2. Always adopt ethical principles and maintain proper etiquette in dealings with patients, relatives and other health personnel and to respect the rights of the patient including the right to information and second opinion.
3. Develop communication skills to word reports and professional opinion as well as to interact with patients, relatives, peers and paramedical staff, and for effective teaching.

C. PSYCHOMOTOR DOMAIN

At the end of the course, the student should acquire following clinical skills and be able to:
1. Interview the patient, elicit relevant and correct information and describe the history in chronological order.
2. Conduct clinical examination, elicit and interpret clinical findings and diagnose common pulmonary disorders and emergencies.
3. Perform simple, routine investigative and office procedures required for making the bedside diagnosis, especially sputum collection and examination for etiologic organisms especially acid fast bacilli (AFB), interpretation of the chest x-rays and lung function tests.
4. Interpret and manage various blood gases abnormalities in various pulmonary
Diseases.
5. Develop management plans for various pulmonary diseases.
6. Assist in the performance of common procedures, like bronchoscopic examination, pleural aspiration and biopsy, pulmonary physiotherapy, endotracheal intubation and pneumo-thoracic drainage / aspiration etc.
7. Recognize emergency situations in intensive care, respond to these appropriately and perform basic critical care monitoring and therapeutic procedures.
8. Collect, compile, analyse, interpret, discuss and present research data.
9. Teach pulmonary medicine to undergraduate and postgraduate students.

To acquire the above skills, the student should be exposed and trained in the following tests and procedures:
1. Diagnostic tests: Performance and interpretation
   - ☐ Sputum and other body fluids examination with ZN stain for AFB, culture methods for pathogenic bacteria, fungi and viruses
   - ☐ Newer diagnostic techniques for tuberculosis including molecular techniques
   - ☐ FNAC of lung masses (blind and image-guided)
   - ☐ Arterial blood gas analysis and pulse oximetry

- ➤ ☐ Imaging: Interpretation of plain radiography, ultrasound examination, Computed tomogram, PET scan, MRI
- ➤ ☐ Sputum cytology
- ➤ ☐ Simple haematological tests
- ➤ ☐ Immunological and Serological tests
- ➤ ☐ Polysomnography (full-night and split-night studies) including CPAP titration; evaluation of daytime sleepiness
- ➤ ☐ Cardiopulmonary exercise testing
- ➤ ☐ Pulmonary function tests and interpretation (Spirometry, lung volume diffusions, body plethysmography, other lung function tests)
- ➤ ☐ Bronchoprovocation tests
- ➤ ☐ BCG vaccination
- ➤ ☐ Mantoux testing; interferon gamma release assays
- ➤ ☐ Bronchoscopy: fibreoptic/rigid, diagnostic and therapeutic
- ➤ ☐ ECG, 2D and Doppler echocardiography
- ➤ ☐ Venous Doppler ultrasound
- ➤ ☐ Skin tests for hypersensitivity
- ➤ ☐ Sputum induction and non-invasive monitoring of airway inflammation
- ➤ ☐ Medical thoracoscopy

2. Therapeutic procedures
- ➤ ☐ Fine needle aspiration and other guided procedures
- ➤ ☐ Tube thoracostomy
- ➤ ☐ Cardiopulmonary rehabilitation exercises
- ➤ ☐ Postural drainage
- ➤ ☐ Pleural biopsy, lymph node biopsy
- ➤ ☐ Administration of inhalation therapy
- ➤ ☐ Administration of oxygen therapy
- ➤ ☐ Administration of continuous positive airway pressure (CPAP)
- ➤ Bilevel Positive Airway Pressure (BiPAP)
- ➤ ☐ Monitoring and emergency procedures in intensive care

CHAPTER 4. SYLLABUS AS PER NMC (INDIA) CURRICULUM

Course contents:
The student should acquire knowledge in the following:
I. Basic Sciences
A. Anatomy and Histology of Respiratory System
1. Development and Anatomy of Respiratory System
2. Applied embryology of lungs, mediastinum and diaphragm
3. Developmental anomalies
B. Physiology and Biochemistry
1. Assessment of pulmonary functions
2. Control of ventilation; pulmonary mechanics
3. Ventilation, pulmonary blood flow, gas exchange and transport
4. Non-respiratory metabolic functions of lung
5. Principles of electrocardiography
6. Inhalation kinetics and its implication in aerosol therapy, and sputum induction
etc.
7. Acid-base and electrolyte balance
8. Physiology of sleep and its disorders
9. Pulmonary innervation and reflexes
10. Pulmonary defence mechanisms
11. Principles of exercise physiology and testing
12. Physiological changes in pregnancy, high altitude, aging
13. Physiological basis of pulmonary symptoms
C. Microbiology
1. Mycobacterium tuberculosis and other mycobacteria
2. Bacteria causing pulmonary diseases
3. Atypical organisms and respiratory tract infections
4. Anaerobes in pleuropulmonary infections
5. Laboratory diagnosis of non-tubercular infections of respiratory tract
6. Laboratory diagnosis of TB including staining, culture and drug sensitivity testing
7. Virulence and pathogenecity of mycobacteria

8. Respiratory viruses: Viral diseases of the respiratory system and diagnostic
methods
9. Respiratory fungi: (i) Classification of fungal diseases of lung: candidiasis,
Actinomycosis, Nacardiosis, Aspergillosis, Blastomycosis etc. (ii) Laboratory
diagnostic procedures in pulmonary mycosis
10. Opportunistic infections in the immuno-ompromised individuals
11. HIV and AIDS. Virological aspects, immuno-pathogenesis, diagnosis
12. Parasitic lung diseases

D. Pathology
1. Acute and chronic inflammation: Pathogenetic mechanisms in pulmonary diseases
2. Pathology aspects of Tuberculosis
3. Pathology aspects of Pneumonias and bronchopulmonary suppuration
4. Chronic bronchitis and emphysema, asthma, other airway diseases
5. Occupational lung diseases including Pneumoconiosis
6. Interstitial lung diseases including sarcoidosis, connective tissue diseases,
pulmonary vasculitis syndromes, pulmonary eosinphilias
7. Tumours of the lung, mediastinum and pleura

E. Epidemiology
1. Epidemiological terms and their definitions
2. Epidemiological methods
3. Epidemiology of tuberculosis, pneumoconiosis, asthma, lung cancer, COPD and
other pulmonary diseases
4. National Tuberculosis Control Programme and RNTCP; Epidemiological aspects
of BCG
5. Epidemiological aspects of pollution-related pulmonary diseases
6. Research methodology, statistics and study designs

F. Allergy and Immunology

1. Various mechanisms of hypersensitivity reactions seen in pulmonary diseases
2. Diagnostic tests in allergic diseases of lung - in vitro and in vivo tests, bronchial
provocation test
3. Immunology of tuberculosis, Sarcoidosis and other diseases with an
immunological basis of pathogenesis

G. Pharmacology
1. Pharmacology of antimicrobial drugs
2. Pharmacology of antitubercular drugs
3. Pharmacology of antineoplastic and immunosuppressant drugs
4. Bronchodilator and anti-inflammatory drugs used in pulmonary diseases
5. Drugs used in viral, fungal and parasitic infections
6. Other drugs pharmacokinetics and drugs interaction of commonly used drugs in
pulmonary diseases
7. Pharmacovigilance

II. Clinical Pulmonary Medicine
Clinical pulmonary medicine covers the entire range of pulmonary diseases. All aspects of pulmonary diseases including epidemiology, aetiopathogenesis, pathology, clinical features, investigations, differential diagnosis and management are to be covered.

A. Infections
1. Tuberculosis
1. Aetiopathogenesis
2. Diagnostic methods
3. Differential diagnosis
4. Management of pulmonary tuberculosis; RNTCP, DOTS, and DOTS-Plus;
International Standards of TB Care
5. Complications in tuberculosis
6. Tuberculosis in children
7. Geriatric tuberculosis
8. Pleural and pericardial effusion and empyema

9. Mycobacteria other than tuberculosis
10. Extrapulmonary tuberculosis
11. HIV and TB; interactions of antitubercular drugs with antiretrovirals
12. Diabetes mellitus and tuberculosis
13. Management of MDR and XDR tuberculosis
2. Non-tuberculous infections of the lungs
- [ ] Approach to a patient with pulmonary infection
- [ ] Community-acquired pneumonia
- [ ] Hospital-associated pneumonia, ventilator-associated pneumonia
- [ ] Unusual and atypical pneumonias including bacterial, viral, fungal and parasitic and ricketsial, anerobic Bronchiectasis, lung abscess and other pulmonary suppurations
  Acquired immunodeficiency syndrome and opportunistic infections in immuno-compromised host
  Principles governing use of antibiotics in pulmonary infections
  Other pneumonias and parasitic infections, Zoonosis

B. Non-infectious Lung Diseases
3. Immunological disorders
   Immune defence mechanisms of the lung
   Sarcoidosis
   Hypersensitivity pneumonitis and lung involvement
   Eosinophilic pneumonias and tropical eosinophilia
   Pulmonary vasculitides
- [ ] Connective tissue diseases involving the respiratory system
- [ ] Interstitial lung disease of other etiologies
- [ ] Reactions of the interstitial space to injury, drugs
- [ ] Occupational and environmental pulmonary diseases

4. Other non-infectious disorders of the lungs and airways
- [ ] Aspiration and inhalational (non-occupational) diseases of the lung
- [ ] Drug induced pulmonary diseases
- [ ] Bullous lung disease
- [ ] Uncommon pulmonary diseases (metabolic, immunological, unknown etiology), pulmonary haemorrhagic syndromes Other pulmonary diseases of unknown etiology including PLCH, LAM, PAP, alveolar microlithiasis

- Cystic fibrosis and disorders of ciliary motility
- Obesity-related pulmonary disorders
- Upper airways obstruction syndromes
- Occupational lung diseases and pneumoconiosis
- Air-pollution induced diseases, toxic lung and other inhalational injuries
- Health hazards of smoking
- Drug-induced lung diseases

5. Pulmonary Circulatory disorders
- Pulmonary hypertension and cor pulmonale
- Pulmonary edema
- Pulmonary thromboembolic diseases and infarction
- Cardiac problems in a pulmonary patient and pulmonary complications produced by cardiac diseases

6. Obstructive diseases of the lungs
   Asthma including allergic bronchopulmonary aspergillosis, specific allergen immunotherapy and immunomodulation Chronic obstructive lung disease and diseases of small airways Special aspects of management including Long term oxygen therapy, Inhalation therapy and Pulmonary rehabilitation

7. Tumors of the lungs
Comprehensive knowledge of neoplastic and non-neoplastic diseases of lung including epidemiology, natural history, staging, and principles of treatment (medical, surgical, and radiation), Solitary pulmonary nodule

8. Diseases of the mediastinum
Non-neoplastic disorders
Benign and malignant (primary and secondary) neoplasms and cysts

9. Disorders of the pleura
- Pleural dynamics and effusions
- Non-neoplastic and neoplastic pleural diseases
- Pneumothorax
- Pyothorax and broncho-pleural fistula
- Fibrothorax

10. Critical Care Pulmonary Medicine

- Management of emergency problems of different pulmonary diseases
- Adult respiratory distress syndrome
- Respiratory failure in the patient with obstructive airway disease
- Respiratory failure in other pulmonary diseases
- Management of sepsis
- Respiratory and haemodynamic monitoring in acute respiratory failure
- Non-invasive and Mechanical ventilation
- Principles of critical care, diagnosis and management of complications;
     severity of illness scoring systems
- Ethical and end-of-life issues in critical care

11. Extrapulmonary manifestations of pulmonary diseases
12. Sleep-related pulmonary diseases
- Polysomnography
- Sleep apneas
- Other sleep-disordered breathing syndromes

13. Miscellaneous aspects
- Diseases of the diaphragm
- Disorders of chest wall
- Obesity-related pulmonary disorders
- Oxygen therapy
- End-of-life care
- Aerospace Medicine
- Pulmonary problems related to special environments (high altitude, diving, miners)
- Assessment of quality of life using questionnaires
- Health impacts of global warming

14. Preventive Pulmonology
- Principles of smoking cessation and smoking cessation strategies
- Cardiopulmonary rehabilitation
- Preventive aspects of pulmonary diseases
- Vaccination in pulmonary diseases

III. Surgical aspects of Pulmonary Medicine

☐ Pre- and post-operative evaluation and management of thoracic surgical patients
☐ Chest trauma/trauma related lung dysfunction
☐ Lung transplantation

CHAPTER 5. TEACHING AND LEARNING METHODS

Postgraduate teaching programme

General principles

Acquisition of practical competencies being the keystone of PG medical education, PG training should be skills oriented. Learning in PG program should be essentially self directed and primarily emanating from clinical and academic work. The formal sessions are merely meant to supplement this core effort.

Teaching methodology

This should include regular bedside case presentations and demonstrations, didactic lectures, seminars, journal clubs, clinical meetings, and combined conferences with allied departments. The post graduate student should be given the responsibility of managing and caring for patients in a gradual manner under supervision.

Formal teaching sessions

In addition to bedside teaching rounds, at least 5-hr of formal teaching per week are necessary. The departments may select a mix of the sessions, as given under formative assessment. Further, the student should:

• Attend accredited scientific meetings (CME, symposia, and conferences).
• Attend additional sessions on resuscitation, basic sciences, biostatistics, research
methodology, teaching methodology, hospital waste management, health economics, medical ethics and legal issues related to medical practice are suggested.
• There should be a training program on Research methodology for existing faculty to build capacity to guide research.
• The postgraduate students shall be required to participate in the teaching and training programme of undergraduate students and interns.
• A postgraduate student of a postgraduate degree course in broad specialities/super specialities would be required to present one poster presentation, to read onepaper at a national/state conference and to

present one research paper which should be published/accepted for publication/sent for publication during the period of his postgraduate studies so as to make him eligible to appear at the postgraduate degree examination.
- Log book: During the training period, the post graduate student should maintain a Log Book indicating the duration of the postings/work done in Wards, OPDs and Casualty. This should indicate the procedures assisted and performed, and the teaching sessions attended. The Log book shall be checked and assessed periodically by the faculty members imparting the training.
- Department should encourage e-learning activities.

THESIS

All MD (Pulmonary Medicine) post graduate students should carry out work on an assigned topic under the direct guidance of a recognised post graduate teacher. A written protocol of the proposed work should be submitted before the end of the first 6 months.

Subsequently, the post graduate student should carry out the proposed work for at least 1 year (not inclusive of the period for submitting the protocol and writing-up the final thesis). During the training programme, patient safety is of paramount importance; therefore, skills are to be learnt initially on the models, later to be performed under supervision followed by performing independently. For this purpose, provision of skills laboratories in medical colleges is mandatory.

ASSESSMENT

FORMATIVE ASSESSMENT, ie., assessment during training. Formative assessment should be continual and should assess medical knowledge patient care, procedural & academic skills, interpersonal skills, professionalism, self directed learning and ability to practice in the system.

General Principles

Internal Assessment should be frequent, cover all domains of learning and used to provide feedback to improve learning; it should also cover professionalism and communication skills. The Internal Assessment should be conducted in theory and practical/clinical examination.

Quarterly assessment during the MD training should be based on:
1. Journal based / recent advances learning
2. Patient based /Laboratory or Skill based learning
3. Self directed learning and teaching
4. Departmental and interdepartmental learning activity
5. External and Outreach Activities / CMEs

The student to be assessed periodically as per categories listed in postgraduate
student appraisal form (as per Annexure I NMC guidance)

SUMMATIVE ASSESSMENT, ie., assessment at the end of training

The summative examination would be carried out as per the Rules given in POSTGRADUATE MEDICAL EDUCATION REGULATIONS, 2000. The Post Graduate Examination shall be in three parts:

1. Thesis:
Every post graduate student shall carry out work on an assigned research project under the guidance of a recognised Post Graduate Teacher, the result of which shall be written up and submitted in the form of a Thesis. Work for writing the Thesis is aimed at contributing to the development of a spirit of enquiry, besides exposing the post graduate student to the techniques of research, critical analysis, acquaintance with the latest advances in medical science and the manner of identifying and consulting available literature. Thesis shall be submitted at least six months before the Theory and Clinical / Practical examination. The thesis shall be examined by a minimum of three examiners; one internal and two external examiners, who shall not be the examiners for Theory and Clinical examination. A post graduate student shall be allowed to appear for the Theory and Practical/Clinical examination only after the acceptance of the Thesis by the examiners.

2. Theory Examination:

The examinations shall be organised on the basis of 'Grading'or 'Marking system' to evaluate and to certify post graduate student's level of knowledge, skill and competence at the end of the training. Obtaining a minimum of 50% marks in 'Theory' as well as 'Practical' *separately* shall be mandatory for passing examination as a whole. The examination for M.D./ MS shall be held at the end of 3rd academic year. An academic term shall mean six month's training period. There shall be four theory papers:

Paper I:	General pulmonary medicine and basic sciences;
Paper II:	Clinical pulmonary medicine including medical emergencies;
Paper III:	Clinical pulmonary medicine including critical care medicine;
Paper IV:	Recent advances in pulmonary medicine, and research methodology.

The final qualifying examination should include an assessment of clinical skills in the form of case presentations and discussions. Other rules laid down by the MCI regarding M.D. examinations shall apply here as well.

3. Practical/Clinical and Oral/viva voce Examination:

The post graduate students shall examine a minimum of **one long and two short cases.**

Oral/viva voce Examination

The oral examination shall be thorough and shall aim at assessing the knowledge and competence of the post graduate student on the subject, investigative procedures, therapeutic technique and other aspects of the specialty which form a part of the examination.

CHAPTER 6; RECOMMENDED BOOKS
'Our eyes cannot see what the Brain doesn't Know'

The phrase "Our eyes cannot see what the brain doesn't know" reflects a fundamental concept in neuroscience and psychology: perception is shaped by prior knowledge and experience. This idea highlights that while our eyes may receive visual input, the brain plays a crucial role in interpreting and making sense of that information. Here's an explanation:

1. Visual Perception Depends on Interpretation

- The retina in the eye captures light and converts it into electrical signals, but these signals are meaningless until processed by the brain.
- The brain uses past experiences, knowledge, and context to interpret what we see. Without these references, the brain might not recognize or make sense of unfamiliar patterns.

Example:

- A person unfamiliar with written language will see letters as meaningless shapes, while a literate person sees them as symbols with meaning.

2. Top-Down Processing

- This refers to the brain's use of existing knowledge and expectations to interpret sensory input.
- If the brain has no prior knowledge or context about an object or situation, it may fail to perceive it correctly, even if the eyes capture the information accurately.

Example:

- Optical illusions or abstract art often confuse the brain because it struggles to apply familiar patterns or logic.

3. Selective Attention and Focus

- The brain filters out unnecessary details to focus on relevant information.
- If the brain doesn't "know" what to look for, important details may be ignored or overlooked.

Example:

- In a radiology scan, an untrained eye may not see subtle abnormalities that a radiologist, with knowledge and training, would immediately identify.

4. Learning Shapes Perception

- The ability to perceive certain objects, colors, or patterns improves with training and experience.
- In unfamiliar environments, individuals may fail to "see" or recognize objects without prior exposure or learning.

Example:

- A person who has never seen a certain type of tool may not recognize its purpose when shown.

5. Neurological Basis

- The visual cortex in the brain integrates visual input with stored memories and concepts.
- Conditions such as visual agnosia (inability to recognize objects despite intact vision) occur when the brain's

knowledge database is disrupted, underscoring the reliance on prior knowledge for perception.

Real-World Implications

1. Education and Training: Training improves the brain's ability to "see" what is important, whether it's recognizing signs of illness in medical imaging or spotting wildlife in nature.
2. Awareness of Biases: The brain's reliance on past knowledge can lead to biases, affecting what we notice or ignore.
3. Art and Creativity: Artists exploit this concept by creating works that challenge our brain's expectations, encouraging new ways of seeing.

In a medical context, the phrase "Our eyes cannot see what the brain doesn't know" is particularly relevant to clinical observation, diagnosis, and interpretation of findings. It underscores the importance of knowledge, training, and experience in medical practice, as they enable a doctor to recognize subtle signs, patterns, and abnormalities that might otherwise go unnoticed.

APPLICATIONS IN MEDICINE

1. Clinical Diagnosis

- A doctor's ability to identify signs of disease is heavily dependent on their knowledge and experience.
- Without prior knowledge of specific disease presentations, a doctor might miss critical diagnostic clues.

Example:

- A novice clinician may see a rash as non-specific, while a dermatologist recognizes it as psoriatic plaques or dermatitis herpetiformis, based on training.

2. Radiology and Imaging

- Radiologists are trained to interpret subtle variations in imaging that indicate pathology.
- Without knowledge of normal anatomy and disease-specific findings, abnormalities may be missed.

Example:

- A small lung nodule might go unnoticed by an untrained observer, while a radiologist identifies it as a potential early-stage carcinoma.

3. Surgery

- During surgery, a surgeon must distinguish between normal and abnormal tissue structures.
- Without a detailed mental "map" of anatomical variations and pathological appearances, errors or oversights could occur.

Example:

- Identifying an inflamed appendix versus nearby mesenteric fat requires a clear understanding of normal anatomy.

4. Pathology

- Pathologists depend on their knowledge of histological patterns to identify abnormalities in tissue biopsies.
- If the brain doesn't "know" how cancer cells look under a microscope, they might be missed.

Example:

- Recognizing Reed-Sternberg cells in Hodgkin's lymphoma requires prior knowledge of their characteristic appearance.

5. Neurology

- A neurologist's ability to recognize subtle neurological deficits relies on understanding how different lesions manifest clinically.

Example:

- The presence of a Babinski sign may be overlooked by a non-specialist but is a critical finding for a neurologist, indicating an upper motor neuron lesion.

6. Emergency Medicine

- In emergency settings, quick and accurate interpretation of visual and clinical cues can save lives.

Example:

- Recognizing cyanosis as a sign of hypoxia or central chest pulsations as indicative of an aortic aneurysm requires prior clinical knowledge.

Importance of Training and Experience

Medical Education:

- Doctors are trained to associate visual cues and clinical findings with specific diseases.
- Anatomy, pathology, and clinical case studies provide the mental framework necessary for accurate diagnosis.

Experience:

- Repeated exposure to clinical cases refines a doctor's ability to "see" patterns and outliers.
- Senior doctors often identify rare conditions simply because they've encountered them before.

Specialization:

- Specialists are more adept at recognizing subtleties in their field because their brain is "primed" to identify them.
- A cardiologist sees subtle ECG changes that might not stand out to a generalist.

Challenges in Medical Practice

Cognitive Biases:

- Relying on prior knowledge can lead to confirmation bias, where a doctor sees what they expect rather than what is present.

Learning Curve:

- New or rare diseases require updating the "mental database" continuously, as diseases evolve or present atypically.

Technology Dependency:

- Over-reliance on diagnostic tools (e.g., AI, imaging software) without understanding the fundamentals can
- limit diagnostic acumen.

SUMMARY

In medicine, a doctor's brain acts as a filter and interpreter for what the eyes see. Continuous learning, experience, and reflection are critical to "knowing" what to look for, allowing the doctor to provide accurate and timely diagnoses. This principle highlights the importance of lifelong learning and clinical exposure in medical practice.

BOOKS (LATEST EDITION); ALWAYS FOLLOW STANDARD BOOKS

1. Harrison's Principles of Internal Medicine ed. Petersdorf (McGraw Hill)
2. Cecil Text book of Medicine ed. Wyngaarden
3. Crofton & Douglas Respiratory diseases ed. Seaton et al (Oxford)
4. Pulmonary diseases & disorders by Fishman (McGraw Hill)
5. Textbook on Pulmonary disease by Fraser & Pare
6. Asthma by Clarke et al
7. Bronchoscopy by Straddling
8. Tuberculosis by SK Sharma
9. Lung diseases in the Tropics ed. OP Sharma (Marcel Dekker)
10. The Normal Lung by Murray (Saunders)
11. Pulmonary Function Testing by Clausen (Academic Press)
12. Respiratory Physiology by J.B. West (Williams & Wilkins)
13. Physiology of Respiration by J.H. Comroe (Yearbook Med Pub.)
14. Respiratory Function in disease by Bates et al (Saunders)

Journals
03-05 international Journals and 02 national (all indexed) journals
NEJM, BTS, Lung India, IJT, ATS

CHAPTER 7; STANDARD PULMONARY DISEASE DEFINITIONS

Standard definitions of pulmonary diseases are crucial in medicine because they ensure consistency, clarity, and reliability in diagnosis, research, and treatment. These standardized definitions are established by authoritative bodies like the American Thoracic Society (ATS), Global Initiative for Chronic Obstructive Lung Disease (GOLD), and others. Here's an overview of their importance:

1. Consistency in Diagnosis

- Standard definitions ensure that clinicians worldwide diagnose pulmonary diseases based on uniform criteria.
- This reduces variability caused by subjective interpretations and enhances diagnostic accuracy.

Example:

- Chronic Obstructive Pulmonary Disease (COPD) is defined by persistent airflow limitation confirmed by spirometry ($FEV_1/FVC < 0.7$). Without this, cases might be over- or under-diagnosed.

2. Facilitation of Research and Comparability

- Standardized definitions allow researchers to study diseases using the same criteria, enabling comparisons across studies and populations.
- This improves the reliability of clinical trials and epidemiological data.

Example:

- The GOLD classification of COPD severity (mild, moderate, severe, very severe) enables researchers to stratify patients and compare outcomes globally.

3. Development of Guidelines and Protocols

- Guidelines like those from GOLD for COPD or GINA for Asthma rely on standard definitions to recommend treatment protocols.
- This ensures treatments are evidence-based and consistent across healthcare systems.

Example:

- Asthma is defined based on variable airflow obstruction and symptoms (wheezing, dyspnea). This standard guides stepwise management in clinical practice.

4. Improved Communication Among Clinicians

- Standardized terminology ensures that doctors, researchers, and policymakers understand each other when discussing pulmonary diseases.
- This is vital for multidisciplinary care and during transitions of care.

Example:

- Using terms like Acute Respiratory Distress Syndrome (ARDS) with its Berlin Definition criteria (PaO_2/FiO_2 ratio, timing, and imaging) ensures uniform communication about severity and prognosis.

5. Public Health and Epidemiology

- Public health interventions require accurate data on disease prevalence and burden, which depends on standardized definitions.
- This allows policymakers to allocate resources effectively.

Example:

- The WHO's definition of tuberculosis includes criteria for pulmonary vs. extrapulmonary TB, enabling precise tracking and intervention planning.

6. Accurate Patient Stratification

- Standardized definitions help stratify patients for tailored treatment and monitoring.
- It ensures patients are appropriately categorized into disease stages or subtypes.

Example:

- In interstitial lung diseases (ILDs), differentiating between idiopathic pulmonary fibrosis (IPF) and hypersensitivity pneumonitis is critical for prognosis and treatment, made possible by standard definitions.

7. Facilitation of Medical Education

- Uniform definitions are essential for training medical professionals, ensuring they learn consistent criteria and approaches.

Example:

- Medical students and trainees are taught to identify pneumonia based on standard clinical features (fever, cough, infiltrates on chest X-ray).

8. Foundation for Advances in Medicine

- Innovations in diagnostics, biomarkers, and treatments rely on clear disease definitions to identify patient populations and measure outcomes effectively.

Example:

- Research into biologic therapies for asthma targets subgroups with high eosinophilic counts, identified using standardized asthma definitions.

Challenges Without Standard Definitions

- Misdiagnosis and inappropriate treatments.
- Difficulty comparing research findings or clinical outcomes.
- Ineffective communication between healthcare providers and researchers.

Standard diseases definition in pulmonary medicine;

ASTHMA
-Asthma is a disease with many variation (Heterogeneous), usually characterize by chronic airflow limitation. It has two key defining features;
1. A history of respiratory symptoms such as cough, wheezing or chest tightness,shortness of breath ,that varies markedly over time AND
2. Variable expiratory flow limitation. ..... GINA 2015
-Asthma is a syndrome characterized by airflow obstruction that varies markedly, both spontaneously and with treatment. ....HPIM

CHRONIC OBSTRUCTIVE PULMONARY DISEASE

-COPD, is common preventable and treatable disease, is characterized by chronic airflow limitation that is usually progressive and associated with enhanced chronic inflammatory response in the airways and the lungs to noxious particle and gases. Exacerbation and co morbidity contribute to overall severity in individual patients.
................GOLD

-COPD, is a disease state characterized by airflow limitation that is not fully reversible.
.........HPIM

ACUTE EXACERBATION OF COPD
-Is defined as acute event characterized by worsening of patient's respiratory symptoms that is beyond normal day to day variation and leads to change in medication.

BRONCHIECTASIS

-Bronchiectasis is an abnormal and permanent dilatation and destruction of bronchi and bronchioles.
...........HPIM

-Bronchiectasis (*broncos,* airways; *ectasia,* dilatation) is a morphologic term used to describe abnormal, irreversibly dilated and thick-walled bronchi. Bronchiectasis represents the end stage of a variety of pathologic processes that cause destruction of the bronchial wall and its surrounding Supporting tissues.
..............Fishman

LUNG ABSCESS
-Lung abscess is defined as pulmonary parenchymal necrosis and cavitations resulting from infection

PNEUMONIA
-Pneumonia is an infection of the pulmonary parenchyma.
-When the word 'pneumonia' is used in medical practice, it almost always refers to a syndrome caused by acute infection, Usually bacterial, characterized by clinical and/or radiographic signs of consolidation of a part or parts of one or both lungs...
.....................Croftan

PNEUMONITIS-
-Pneumonitis is occasionally used as a synonym for pneumonia, particularly when inflammation of the lung has resulted from a *non-infectious cause, such as chemical or radiation injury*.
.... Crofton

CYSTIC FIBROSIS-
-Cystic fibrosis (CF) is a monogenic disorder that presents as a multisystem disease.

ILD(Interstitial Lung Disease)
-ILDs represent a large number of conditions that involve the parenchyma of the lung—the alveoli, the alveolar epithelium, the capillary endothelium, and the spaces between these structures, as well as the perivascular and lymphatic tissues

EMPYEMA-

-The word 'empyema' is used to denote the presence of pus in a natural body cavity. In respiratory medicine that space is the pleural cavity and the term is often also used to cover pus in a postpneumonectomy space...   ...Croftan
-An empyema, by definition is pus in the pleural space.
-Weese et al. (32) defined an empyema as pleural fluid with a specific gravity greater than 1 .018, a WBC count greater than 500 cells/mm3, or a protein level greater than 2 . 5 g/dL

-Vianna (33) defined an empyema as pleural fluid on which the bacterial cultures are positive or the WBC is greater than 1 5 ,000/ mm3 and the protein level is above 3.0 g/dL.

OBSTRUCTIVE SLEEP APNEA(OSA)
-OSAHS may be defined as the coexistence of unexplained excessive daytime sleepiness with at least five obstructed breathing events (apnea or hypopnea) per hour of sleep.

-*Apneas* are defined in adults as breathing pauses lasting ≥10 s.

-hypopneas as ≥10 s during which there is continued breathing but the ventilation is reduced by at least 50% from the previous baseline during sleep ...
...(HPIM)

SOLITARY PULMONARY NODULES;

-Solitary pulmonary nodule (SPN) refers to a single, focal, round or ovoid lesion of the lung parenchyma measuring up to 3 cm in the diameter detected on chest X-ray *without* any associated adenopathy, atelectasis or Consolidation.

-If the size is more than 3 cm it is referred as **mass lesion.**

ANEMIA-
-According to the World Health Organization (WHO), anemia is defined as a hemoglobin level of less than 13 g/dL in men and less than 12 g/dL in women

-According to the World Health Organization (WHO), anemia is defined as a hemoglobin level of less than 13 g/dL in men and less than 12 g/dL in women

CHRONIC BRONCHITIS-

-Chronic bronchitis is a condition characterized by cough with or without expectoration on most of the days in a week for at least 3 months in a year for 2 consecutive years (WHO).

EMPHYSEMA
-Emphysema is characterized by *abnormal permanent enlargement of the airspaces* distal to the terminal bronchioles, accompanied by *destruction of their walls* without obvious fibrosis.

OVERINFLATION-
Enlargement of airspaces is not accompanied by destruction; this is more correctly called *overinflation*.

A second-line TB drug: This is an agent reserved for the treatment of drug-resistant TB. First-line TB drugs used to treat drug-susceptible TB – ethambutol, isoniazid, and pyrazinamide – may also be used in MDR-TB regimens (streptomycin is now considered a second-line TB drug and used only as a substitute for amikacin when amikacin is not available or there is confirmed resistance to it).

Bacteriologically confirmed TB: TB diagnosed in a biological specimen by smear microscopy, culture, or a WHO-endorsed rapid molecular test adopted by NTEP.

Disseminated TB: is defined as the presence of two or more noncontiguous sites resulting from hematogenous and/or lymphatic dissemination of *Mycobacterium tuberculosis*, occurring because of progressive primary infection, reactivation of a latent focus with subsequent spread, or rarely through iatrogenic origin. Milliary TB is also a form of disseminated TB

Drug-susceptibility testing: DST refers to in-vitro testing using either of the phenotypic methods to determine susceptibility.

Drug resistance testing: DRT refers to in-vitro testing using genotypic methods (molecular techniques) to determine resistance.

Extensively drug-resistant TB (XDR-TB): TB caused by M.tb strains that fulfil the definition of MDR/RR-TB and are also resistant to any fluoroquinolone (levofloxacin or moxifloxacin) and at least one additional Group A drug (presently to either bedaquiline or linezolid [or both].

Extensive or severe form of TB: Extensive TB disease includes presence of bilateral cavitary disease or extensive parenchymal damage on chest radiography & in children aged under 15 years, presence of cavity or bilateral disease on chest radiography. Severe EP-TB disease includes presence of *TB-meningitis, or CNS TB, spinal/ skeletal TB, or disseminated TB (miliary TB or TB with multiorgan involvement).* Severe EP-TB disease includes in children aged under 15 years, extrapulmonary forms of disease other than pleural effusion & lymphadenopathy (peripheral nodes or isolated mediastinal mass without compression). In children, the occurrence of advanced malnutrition (defined by syndrome or by metrics) or advanced immunosuppression or positive tuberculosis (TB) bacteriology (smear, NAAT, culture) may also be considered when determining disease severity.

Isoniazid-resistant TB (Hr-TB): TB is caused by M.tb strains that are resistant to isoniazid, and susceptibility to rifampicin has been confirmed.

Mono-resistant TB (MR TB): TB caused by M.tb strains that are resistant to one first- line anti-TB drug only.

Multidrug-resistant TB (MDR-TB): TB caused by M.tb strains that are resistant to both H and R with or without resistance to other first-line anti-TB drugs. MDR-TB patients may have additional resistance to any/all FQ or any other second-line anti-TB drug.

Presumptive TB: This refers to a person with any of the symptoms, signs or chest X-ray abnormality.

Presumptive DR-TB: It refers to the patient who is eligible for rifampicin-resistant screening at the time of diagnosis OR/and during treatment for DS-TB or H mono/poly DR-TB. [This includes all notified TB patients (Public and private), follow-up positive on microscopy including treatment failures on standard first- line treatment and H mono/poly DR-TB regimen and any clinical non-responder, including paediatric].

Pre-extensively drug-resistant TB (Pre-XDR-TB): TB caused by M.tb strains that fulfil the definition of MDR/ RR-TB and are also resistant to any fluoroquinolone.

Poly-drug resistant TB (PDR-TB): TB caused by M.tb strains that are resistant to more than one first-line anti-TB drug other than H and R.

Rifampicin resistant TB (RR-TB): TB caused by M.tb strains that are resistant to R, detected using phenotypic or genotypic methods, with or without resistance to other anti-TB drugs. Itincludes any resistance to R in the form of mono-resistance, poly-resistance, MDR-TB, orXDR-TB.

Serious adverse events: SAEs are those adverse events (AEs) classified as Grade 3 (severe), Grade 4 (life-threatening or disabling) or Grade 5 (death related to AE) or which led to the drug being stopped permanently. SAEs are otherwise often defined as AEs that either leads to death or a life-threatening experience; to initial or prolonged hospitalization; to persistent or significant disability; or to a congenital anomaly. The management of SAEs may require the termination of the drug suspected of having caused the event.

Universal DST: Refers to universal access to rapid DRT for at least rifampicin and furtherDST/DRT for at least fluoroquinolones among all TB patients with rifampicin resistance(preferably before initiation of treatment to a maximum within 15 days of diagnosis).

Obstructive airway Disease (OAD)-Obstructive airway disease is a condition characterized by a reduction in airflow due to partial or complete obstruction of the airways, which leads to difficulty in exhaling air from the lungs.

SUMMARY

Standard pulmonary disease definitions are indispensable for clinical care, research, and public health. They ensure that patients receive the correct diagnosis and treatment while enabling global collaboration to improve pulmonary health. Adopting and adhering to these standards is a cornerstone of evidence-based medical practice.

CHAPTER 8; HOW TO LEARN IN MD PULMONARY MEDICINE RESIDENCY DESPITE A HECTIC WORK SCHEDULE

Residency in Pulmonary Medicine is both challenging and rewarding. The demanding schedule often leaves little time for structured learning, but with proper strategies, you can optimize your education even amidst a busy workload. This chapter provides actionable steps to help residents learn effectively during their training.

1. Adopt a Mindset of Continuous Learning

- Integrate Learning into Daily Tasks: View every patient encounter as an opportunity to learn. Focus on understanding the underlying pathology, differential diagnoses, and management plans. Ask yourself, "What can I learn from this case?"
- Be Curious: Actively seek answers to questions that arise during rounds or procedures. Use downtime to quickly read about topics you encounter.

2. Set Realistic Learning Goals

- Daily Goals: Identify one or two key topics to review each day, such as a pulmonary condition, diagnostic method, or treatment approach.
- Weekly Goals: Choose a specific area to focus on each week, like interpreting pulmonary function tests (PFTs) or reviewing the management of COPD exacerbations.

3. Use Short and High-Yield Resources

- Apps and Online Tools: Use resources like UpToDate, Medscape, and PubMed for quick, evidence-based information.

- Videos and Podcasts: Platforms like YouTube (e.g., *medeasy 2023@wi7ni*, Dr. Najeeb's Lectures) or podcasts such as The Curbsiders offer concise and engaging ways to learn.
- Flashcards: Use apps like Anki to review key concepts and retain facts through spaced repetition.

4. Master Bedside Learning

- Case-Based Learning: Discuss cases with attendings and peers to understand their approach to diagnosis and management.
- Procedural Learning: During bronchoscopy, thoracentesis, or other procedures, focus on both the technical skills and the rationale behind the intervention.
- Clinical Question Journal: Maintain a notebook or digital file where you jot down unanswered questions during the day and follow up later.

5. Leverage Morning Rounds and Conferences

- Actively Participate: Engage in discussions during rounds, ask relevant questions, and take notes.
- Utilize Teaching Moments: Many programs include mini-lectures during rounds or morning conferences. Be attentive and review the material later.

6. Time Management Techniques

- Prioritize Learning Opportunities: Focus on high-yield areas like managing acute conditions (e.g., ARDS, asthma exacerbations) and interpreting imaging studies.
- Block Study Time: Dedicate 15-30 minutes of focused study during quieter periods, such as early mornings or between shifts.
- Pomodoro Technique: Use short, focused intervals (e.g., 25 minutes) for studying with breaks in between.

7. Collaborate with Peers

- Study Groups: Partner with fellow residents to review challenging topics or cases.
- Peer Teaching: Explaining concepts to peers reinforces your understanding and helps identify knowledge gaps.

8. Optimize Learning During Procedures and Clinics

- Ask Questions: Inquire about techniques, indications, and complications during procedures.
- Reflect on Cases: After clinic sessions, review cases seen that day, focusing on diagnostic dilemmas and management strategies.

9. Utilize Technology

- Digital Notes: Use apps like Notion, Evernote, or Google Keep to organize learning materials.
- Clinical Guidelines Apps: Keep guidelines such as GOLD for COPD or ATS/ERS for ILD readily accessible on your phone.

10. Prepare for Exams Gradually

- Cumulative Learning: Avoid cramming. Incorporate board review questions into daily learning to build knowledge incrementally.
- Review Past Cases: Use your own clinical experiences to anchor theoretical knowledge.

11. Seek Feedback and Mentorship

- Ask for Feedback: Regularly request feedback from attendings to identify areas for improvement.
- Mentorship: Find a mentor who can guide your academic growth and clinical skills development.

12. Maintain Work-Life Balance

- Self-Care: Ensure adequate sleep, nutrition, and exercise to maintain focus and prevent burnout.
- Mindfulness: Practice mindfulness or relaxation techniques to manage stress and improve mental clarity.

13. Reflect and Adapt

- End-of-Day Reflection: Spend 5-10 minutes at the end of each day reflecting on what you learned and areas to improve.
- Adapt Strategies: Regularly evaluate your learning methods and adjust them to fit your needs and schedule.

SUMMARY

Despite the challenges of a demanding residency schedule, adopting effective learning strategies can help you grow as a competent pulmonologist. By integrating learning into daily tasks, using high-yield resources, and leveraging available opportunities, you can make consistent progress while managing the workload of residency.

CHAPTER 9; ETHICAL AND HUMANITARIAN IMPLICATIONS OF POOR TRAINING IN MD PULMONARY MEDICINE RESIDENCY IN THE INDIAN CONTEXT

The quality of training in MD Pulmonary Medicine residency programs has profound ethical and humanitarian implications. In the Indian context, where the burden of pulmonary diseases such as tuberculosis (TB), chronic obstructive pulmonary disease (COPD), asthma, and environmental lung diseases is substantial, inadequate training can have far-reaching consequences for patients, healthcare systems, and society. This chapter explores these implications in detail.

1. Impact on Patient Care

1.1. Increased Morbidity and Mortality

- Poorly trained pulmonologists may lack the skills to diagnose and manage life-threatening conditions such as acute respiratory distress syndrome (ARDS), severe asthma exacerbations, or advanced-stage lung cancer.
- Delay in recognizing critical conditions like multidrug-resistant tuberculosis (MDR-TB) can lead to worsening patient outcomes and higher mortality rates.

1.2. Misdiagnosis and Overdiagnosis

- Inadequate training in diagnostic techniques such as pulmonary function tests (PFTs), bronchoscopy, and imaging may lead to errors. For example:
    - Misdiagnosing lung cancer as tuberculosis can delay appropriate care.

- Overdiagnosis of asthma or COPD may result in unnecessary treatment and medication-related side effects.

1.3. Compromised Procedural Skills

- Lack of hands-on training in procedures like thoracentesis, bronchoscopy, or pleural biopsy increases the risk of complications, leading to patient harm and potential legal liability.

2. Ethical Issues

2.1. Breach of Professional Responsibility

- Physicians have a moral duty to provide competent care. Substandard training undermines this obligation, violating the ethical principle of beneficence (acting in the best interest of patients).

2.2. Loss of Patient Trust

- Poor clinical outcomes erode trust in physicians and the healthcare system, particularly in rural or underserved areas where access to pulmonologists is already limited.

2.3. Resource Wastage

- Mismanagement of pulmonary conditions leads to wasted healthcare resources, which is especially unethical in a resource-constrained country like India.

3. Humanitarian Consequences

3.1. Widening Health Disparities

- Poorly trained doctors disproportionately affect marginalized populations, worsening health inequities. For instance:
  - Rural patients, who rely heavily on government healthcare facilities, are more vulnerable to receiving inadequate care.
  - Delay in managing conditions like TB in these populations can lead to widespread community transmission.

3.2. Public Health Impact

- Inadequate training in recognizing and managing environmental and occupational lung diseases may result in underreporting and poor prevention strategies.
- Failure to control infectious diseases like TB exacerbates India's public health crisis.

3.3. Psychological Toll on Patients

- Mismanagement or prolonged suffering due to poor diagnosis and treatment causes emotional and financial distress for patients and their families, compounding the humanitarian burden.

4. Systemic Implications

4.1. Compromised Medical Education Standards

- Substandard residency training programs reflect systemic issues in medical education, including:
  - Lack of qualified faculty.
  - Inadequate infrastructure for hands-on training.
  - Overburdened teaching hospitals with insufficient patient-doctor ratios.

4.2. Workforce Inefficiency

- Graduates with inadequate training enter the workforce ill-prepared to manage the complex respiratory diseases prevalent in India, perpetuating a cycle of inefficiency.

4.3. International Reputation

- Poor training standards may affect the credibility of Indian medical education globally, limiting opportunities for collaboration and professional growth.

5. Solutions to Address Training Deficiencies

5.1. Strengthening Residency Programs

- Enhance curriculum standardization across institutions with input from professional bodies like the Indian Chest Society (ICS) and National Medical Commission (NMC).
- Incorporate simulation-based training for procedures and emergency management.

5.2. Faculty Development

- Provide advanced training and workshops for faculty to improve teaching and mentorship skills.
- Incentivize experienced pulmonologists to serve as trainers in underserved regions.

5.3. Infrastructure Investment

- Upgrade diagnostic and procedural facilities in medical colleges to ensure residents gain hands-on experience with modern tools.

5.4. Periodic Assessments and Accreditation

- Implement stringent assessments for residency programs to ensure compliance with quality standards.
- Revoke accreditation for programs failing to meet minimum requirements.

5.5. Ethical Training

- Include medical ethics and communication skills as a core part of the curriculum to ensure holistic patient care.

SUMMARY

Poor training in MD Pulmonary Medicine residency programs has significant ethical and humanitarian implications, especially in the Indian context where the burden of respiratory diseases is immense. Addressing these challenges requires systemic reforms in medical education, infrastructure, and ethical practices. By improving the quality of training, India can ensure that its pulmonologists are equipped to provide competent, compassionate care and uphold the highest standards of medical ethics.

CHAPTER 10; LEGAL IMPLICATIONS OF POOR TRAINING IN MD PULMONARY MEDICINE RESIDENCY IN THE INDIAN CONTEXT

Residency training in Pulmonary Medicine is a crucial phase in producing competent specialists who can manage a wide spectrum of respiratory diseases. However, inadequate or substandard training can lead to serious legal, ethical, and professional implications, especially in India where the healthcare landscape presents unique challenges. This chapter explores the legal ramifications of poor residency training, the accountability of institutions, and measures to mitigate these issues.

1. Understanding Legal Liability in Medical Training

1.1. Duty of Care in Training

- Medical colleges and teaching hospitals have a duty to provide residents with adequate training to ensure they become competent specialists.
- Failure to meet this duty can result in medical negligence claims under the Consumer Protection Act (CPA), 2019, where patients may sue for substandard care resulting from poorly trained doctors.

1.2. Vicarious Liability

- Hospitals and institutions can be held vicariously liable for errors committed by inadequately trained residents, as they are responsible for overseeing their education and supervision.

2. Potential Consequences of Poor Training

2.1. Errors in Patient Care

- Poorly trained residents are more likely to make diagnostic and therapeutic errors, leading to adverse patient outcomes and potential legal action for malpractice.

Example: A resident unable to identify or manage acute respiratory distress syndrome (ARDS) due to inadequate training may face allegations of negligence.

2.2. Breach of Ethical Standards

- Substandard training compromises patient safety, violating ethical principles of non-maleficence (do no harm) and beneficence (act in the patient's best interest).

2.3. Professional Repercussions

- Poorly trained pulmonologists risk facing disciplinary action by medical regulatory bodies like the National Medical Commission (NMC) for professional incompetence.

3. Legal Framework Governing Medical Training in India

3.1. National Medical Commission (NMC) Regulations

- The Postgraduate Medical Education Regulations, 2000, outline the standards for residency training. Institutions failing to meet these standards may face penalties or loss of accreditation.

3.2. Consumer Protection Act (CPA), 2019

- Patients affected by negligence linked to inadequate training can file complaints under the CPA, which includes provisions for compensation for deficiency in services.

3.3. Civil and Criminal Liability

- Errors due to poor training can result in:
    - Civil cases: Seeking monetary compensation for harm caused.
    - Criminal cases: If gross negligence leads to death, charges under Section 304A of the Indian Penal Code (IPC) may apply.

4. Institutional Responsibility

4.1. Ensuring Adequate Training

- Institutions must adhere to NMC guidelines by providing:
    - Competent faculty and infrastructure.
    - Structured clinical exposure and procedural training.
    - Regular evaluations of residents' performance.

4.2. Supervision and Mentorship

- Faculty must supervise residents during critical procedures like bronchoscopy, thoracentesis, and ventilator management to prevent errors and foster learning.

5. Addressing Poor Training Outcomes

5.1. Role of Institutions

- Implement comprehensive training programs focusing on core competencies in pulmonary medicine.
- Ensure regular audits of residency programs to maintain quality.

5.2. Role of Residents

- Residents must actively engage in learning opportunities and report deficiencies in training to program directors or institutional heads.

5.3. Legal Safeguards for Patients

- Institutions should maintain transparency in addressing patient complaints and resolving disputes to mitigate legal risks.

6. Case Studies and Precedents

6.1. Notable Legal Cases

- Cases where medical institutions have been held liable for negligence due to poorly trained doctors underscore the importance of proper training.

Example: In instances of mismanagement of pulmonary diseases like tuberculosis or lung cancer, courts have ordered compensation for harm caused by incorrect treatment.

6.2. Lessons Learned

- These cases highlight the necessity for robust training, regular assessment, and adherence to clinical guidelines.

7. Preventive Measures to Avoid Legal Repercussions

7.1. Strengthening Residency Programs

- Periodic curriculum updates aligned with advancements in pulmonary medicine.
- Incorporation of simulation-based training for procedures.

7.2. Enhancing Faculty Accountability

- Regular training for faculty to improve teaching methods and supervision skills.

7.3. Promoting a Culture of Feedback

- Open channels for residents to provide feedback on training quality and identify gaps.

SUMMARY

The legal implications of poor training in MD Pulmonary Medicine residency are significant, affecting not only patient safety but also the reputation of institutions and the careers of residents. By adhering to regulatory standards, fostering a robust training environment, and ensuring ethical practices, institutions and residents can minimize legal risks and improve healthcare outcomes. Strengthening the residency framework is not just a legal obligation but a moral imperative to ensure the development of competent pulmonologists.

CHAPTER 11; HOW TO ENJOY A MD RESIDENCY PROGRAM DESPITE HECTIC WORK HOURS

Residency is a demanding yet transformative phase of a medical career. While the long hours and high stress levels can feel overwhelming, it's entirely possible to find joy and satisfaction in the journey. This chapter provides practical strategies to balance professional responsibilities with personal fulfillment, making the residency experience enjoyable and meaningful.

1. Adopt a Positive Mindset

1.1. Embrace the Challenge

- Understand that residency is a stepping stone to becoming a skilled physician. Every difficult moment contributes to your growth.
- Remind yourself why you chose this path, focusing on your passion for medicine and helping others.

1.2. Celebrate Small Wins

- Acknowledge and appreciate daily achievements, whether it's mastering a procedure, making a correct diagnosis, or connecting with a patient.
- Share your successes with colleagues, friends, or mentors to boost morale.

2. Cultivate Strong Relationships

2.1. Build Camaraderie with Peers

- Develop friendships with fellow residents who understand your struggles and can provide support.
- Organize group activities such as dinners, outings, or movie nights to unwind together.

2.2. Connect with Mentors

- Seek guidance from faculty or senior residents who can offer perspective and advice.
- Mentors can help you navigate challenges and recognize opportunities for growth.

3. Prioritize Work-Life Balance

3.1. Manage Time Effectively

- Use tools like planners or apps to schedule work, study, and leisure activities.
- Dedicate short, focused periods for studying, and ensure you reserve time for relaxation.

3.2. Make Time for Hobbies

- Pursue interests outside of medicine to recharge your mind. Even 15-30 minutes a day can be rejuvenating.
- Examples include reading, painting, cooking, gardening, or listening to music.

4. Create Moments of Joy During Work

4.1. Build Rapport with Patients

- Engaging with patients on a personal level can make your day more fulfilling.
- A smile, kind words, or listening attentively can create meaningful connections.

4.2. Enjoy Teamwork

- Foster a sense of teamwork by supporting and collaborating with colleagues.

- Humor and light-hearted conversations during breaks can ease stress.

5. Maintain Physical and Mental Health

5.1. Exercise Regularly

- Even short sessions of physical activity, such as yoga, running, or gym workouts, can boost energy and mood.
- Use hospital gyms or take a brisk walk during breaks to stay active.

5.2. Eat Healthy

- Opt for nutritious meals and snacks to maintain energy levels.
- Meal prepping can save time and help avoid unhealthy eating habits.

5.3. Practice Mindfulness and Relaxation

- Engage in activities like meditation, deep breathing, or journaling to manage stress.
- Apps like Calm or Headspace can guide you through mindfulness exercises.

6. Incorporate Fun into Learning

6.1. Gamify Study Sessions

- Use flashcard apps like Anki or play quiz games with peers to make studying enjoyable.
- Turn case discussions into friendly competitions to spark interest.

6.2. Attend Conferences and Workshops

- Participating in medical conferences allows you to network and explore new knowledge in exciting environments.
- Use these events as opportunities for travel and leisure alongside professional growth.

7. Plan and Reward Yourself

7.1. Schedule Breaks

- Plan vacations or weekend getaways to recharge. Even a day off can help reset your mind.
- Explore local attractions or engage in activities you enjoy during your time off.

7.2. Treat Yourself

- Reward yourself with small indulgences like your favorite meal, a movie, or a new gadget after completing a tough rotation.

8. Develop Resilience

8.1. Learn from Challenges

- View setbacks as opportunities to grow rather than as failures.
- Reflect on difficult situations and how they contribute to your development.

8.2. Seek Support When Needed

- Don't hesitate to talk to a counselor, mentor, or trusted friend if you feel overwhelmed.
- Residency programs often have mental health resources—make use of them.

9. Find Purpose and Meaning

9.1. Focus on the Big Picture

- Remember that your work has a profound impact on patients' lives and the community.
- Reflect on your journey and how it aligns with your long-term goals.

9.2. Keep a Gratitude Journal

- Write down moments of gratitude each day, whether it's about a patient's recovery or a kind gesture from a colleague.
- Gratitude helps shift focus from stress to positive experiences.

SUMMARY

Enjoying your MD residency is about finding balance, building relationships, and focusing on growth. By adopting a positive attitude, managing time wisely, and seeking joy in small moments, you can turn this intense phase of training into one of personal and professional fulfillment. Remember, the residency journey is as much about becoming a compassionate and skilled doctor as it is about discovering your resilience and capacity for joy.

CHAPTER 12; IMPORTANCE OF BASIC STATISTICAL KNOWLEDGE IN MD RESIDENCY PROGRAMS

Statistics is the backbone of evidence-based medicine (EBM). For MD residents, a solid understanding of basic statistical principles is crucial not only for interpreting medical literature but also for conducting research, improving patient care, and making informed clinical decisions. This chapter explores why statistical knowledge is essential in residency training and how it enhances the practice of modern medicine.

1. Foundation of Evidence-Based Medicine (EBM)

1.1. Critical Appraisal of Research

- Understanding statistics enables residents to critically evaluate the validity and reliability of clinical studies.
- Skills such as interpreting p-values, confidence intervals, and study designs are essential to assess the strength of evidence.

1.2. Application in Clinical Decision-Making

- Statistics guide decisions on treatment efficacy, risk-benefit analysis, and diagnostic test accuracy.
- Example: Sensitivity, specificity, positive predictive value (PPV), and negative predictive value (NPV) are critical metrics when evaluating diagnostic tests.

2. Enhances Research and Academic Contributions

2.1. Designing Robust Studies

- Basic statistical knowledge helps residents design studies with appropriate methodologies, sample sizes, and statistical tests.

- Understanding concepts like randomization, blinding, and control groups ensures higher-quality research.

2.2. Accurate Data Analysis

- Residents can use statistical tools to analyze their research data effectively, ensuring valid and meaningful SUMMARYs.
- Familiarity with software like SPSS, R, or Microsoft Excel enhances their research capabilities.

2.3. Publication and Presentations

- Accurate statistical interpretation strengthens manuscripts and presentations, increasing the likelihood of acceptance in peer-reviewed journals.
- Residents can confidently present their findings at conferences and contribute to medical knowledge.

3. Improved Patient Care Through Data Interpretation

3.1. Individualized Patient Care

- Statistics aid in understanding population-based data and applying it to individual patients.
- Example: Risk calculators and prediction models often rely on statistical principles.

3.2. Monitoring Outcomes

- Tracking patient outcomes, complication rates, and treatment effectiveness relies on statistical methods.
- Continuous quality improvement projects benefit from sound data analysis.

4. Better Understanding of Public Health

4.1. Epidemiology

- Knowledge of epidemiological statistics helps residents understand disease prevalence, incidence, and distribution.
- Example: Interpreting trends in infectious diseases like tuberculosis or COVID-19.

4.2. Health Policy and Resource Allocation

- Statistics inform resource allocation and policy-making, which residents can influence through evidence-based advocacy.

5. Essential Statistical Concepts for MD Residents

5.1. Descriptive Statistics

- Mean, median, mode, standard deviation, and variance.
- Use: Summarizing patient data or study populations.

5.2. Inferential Statistics

- Hypothesis testing, confidence intervals, and p-values.
- Use: Determining whether study findings are due to chance or are statistically significant.

5.3. Correlation and Regression

- Understanding relationships between variables.
- Use: Exploring predictors of outcomes or trends over time.

5.4. Probability and Risk Assessment

- Absolute risk, relative risk, odds ratio, and number needed to treat (NNT).

- Use: Assessing treatment effectiveness and patient counseling.

5.5. Common Statistical Tests

- t-tests, chi-square tests, ANOVA, and non-parametric tests.
- Use: Comparing groups or analyzing categorical data.

6. Challenges and Solutions

6.1. Barriers to Learning Statistics

- Many residents find statistics intimidating due to its mathematical nature.
- Limited time during residency can make structured learning difficult.

6.2. Overcoming the Barriers

- Integration into Curriculum: Incorporate statistics training into residency programs through workshops and online courses.
- Use of Simplified Tools: Introduce user-friendly software for data analysis.
- Mentorship: Pair residents with statisticians or research mentors for guidance.

7. Practical Tips for Residents

- Start Small: Focus on mastering essential concepts before diving into advanced topics.
- Utilize Resources: Use textbooks, online platforms (e.g., Coursera, Khan Academy), and institutional workshops.
- Practice Regularly: Analyze real data from clinical practice or research to solidify understanding.

- Collaborate: Work with statisticians or peers experienced in data analysis.

SUMMARY

Basic statistical knowledge is an indispensable tool for MD residents. It empowers them to interpret research, contribute to academic medicine, and provide evidence-based care. By integrating statistics into daily practice and learning gradually, residents can overcome challenges and make informed decisions that enhance patient outcomes and their professional growth.

CHAPTER 13: A CODE OF ETHICS AND PROFESSIONAL CONDUCT FOR RESIDENT DOCTORS

1. Introduction

The life of a resident doctor is demanding, requiring dedication, resilience, and a high level of professionalism. It is a period of intense learning and growth, where young doctors transition from students to independent medical practitioners. Alongside academic and clinical proficiency, maintaining personal integrity, ethical standards, and healthy lifestyle choices is crucial. Addiction and poor character can significantly impact not only the individual's career but also the health of patients, the working environment, and the reputation of the medical profession. This chapter outlines the importance of maintaining a drug-free, ethical, and professional life for resident doctors and provides practical guidance on how to achieve this.

2. The Importance of Professional Conduct in Residency

Resident doctors are entrusted with the health and well-being of their patients. They are role models for medical students, interns, and junior staff, and their behavior reflects the values of their institution and the broader medical profession. Any deviation from ethical conduct or engagement in harmful behaviors, such as addiction, can jeopardize patient care and their professional relationships.

Patient Care: A resident doctor's primary responsibility is to deliver the best care to patients. Impaired judgment, lack of concentration, or emotional instability due to addiction or poor character traits can lead to mistakes, misdiagnoses, and compromised care, potentially leading to adverse outcomes.

Peer Influence: Resident doctors are in a highly competitive environment where their conduct shapes the culture of the hospital or medical institution. It is essential to uphold ethical standards to inspire and mentor junior colleagues, creating a positive and supportive atmosphere within the team.

Personal Growth: Residency is a time for personal and professional growth. Maintaining high moral standards and resisting temptations, such as addiction, ensures that the focus remains on learning and developing the skills necessary for a successful medical career.

3. Addiction and Its Impact on Resident Doctors

Addiction, in any form, can have severe consequences for a resident doctor's career and personal life. Whether it involves substance abuse, alcohol dependence, or behavioral addictions (such as gambling or technology addiction), it can impair cognitive function, decision-making, and physical health.

Common Addictions among Resident Doctors:

Substance Abuse (Drugs & Alcohol): The demanding nature of residency, coupled with stress, long hours, and emotional burnout, might tempt some doctors to turn to substances as a coping mechanism. However, substance abuse can severely affect one's ability to think clearly, function efficiently, and manage stressful situations.

Workaholism and Burnout: While not a substance addiction, excessive dedication to work at the expense of personal well-being can be seen as a form of addiction. This can lead to burnout, fatigue, and emotional exhaustion, all of which compromise the quality of care provided to patients and hinder personal development.

Technology Addiction: With the increasing use of smartphones and social media, resident doctors are also at risk of becoming addicted to technology. This addiction can lead to distractions during work hours, negatively affecting performance and relationships with patients and colleagues.

Consequences of Addiction:

- Compromised Clinical Judgment: Addiction impairs cognitive functions such as attention, memory, and decision-making, leading to mistakes that can jeopardize patient care and safety.
- Decreased Physical and Mental Health: Addiction often leads to physical health issues, including liver damage, neurological impairment, and mental health disorders such as depression and anxiety.
- Legal and Professional Consequences: Engaging in substance abuse or other illegal activities can lead to legal consequences, including the loss of medical license, suspension from the residency program, or disqualification from future opportunities in the field.

4. Maintaining a Strong Moral Character

Beyond the avoidance of addiction, maintaining a good character is fundamental to professional success and the trust placed in a resident doctor. A good character encompasses qualities like integrity, honesty, compassion, accountability, and respect for others. Upholding these values is critical for patient safety, professional relationships, and personal satisfaction.

Key Aspects of a Good Character:

1. **Honesty and Transparency**: Resident doctors must be truthful in their clinical decisions, documentation, and communication with patients, their families, and colleagues. Dishonesty, such as falsifying

medical records or making unethical decisions, can severely harm patients and lead to professional consequences.

2. **Accountability and Responsibility**: A resident doctor must take responsibility for their actions, including their mistakes. Being accountable is a crucial aspect of maintaining trust with patients and colleagues. This also means seeking guidance when unsure or needing support, and learning from errors to improve practice.

3. **Compassion and Empathy**: Effective patient care requires more than just medical knowledge—it also requires understanding the emotional and psychological needs of patients. Compassion and empathy are at the heart of patient-centered care and contribute to better patient outcomes and satisfaction.

4. **Respect and Professionalism**: Treating all individuals—patients, staff, and peers—with respect and dignity is a cornerstone of medical practice. Professionalism includes maintaining appropriate boundaries, being punctual, collaborating with colleagues, and adhering to ethical guidelines.

Building and Maintaining Character:

1. **Continuous Self-Reflection**: Engaging in regular self-assessment and reflection is essential for maintaining personal integrity. This helps identify areas for improvement and ensures that personal behaviors align with professional values.

2. **Mentorship and Guidance**: Seeking mentorship from senior doctors or counselors can provide valuable guidance on navigating the stresses of residency while maintaining ethical standards. Mentorship also offers emotional support and practical advice on handling complex situations.

3. **Setting Boundaries and Seeking Support:** Recognizing when to take a break, seek help, or talk to someone about mental or emotional health challenges is vital. Many residency programs offer counseling services or peer support groups to help doctors cope with stress and prevent burnout.

5. **Institutional Support and Policies**

Medical institutions and residency programs should have clear policies in place to support resident doctors in maintaining a drug-free and ethical professional life. These include:

1. **Counseling and Mental Health Resources**: Providing access to mental health resources, counseling services, and stress management programs to support resident doctors in maintaining their well-being.
2. **Wellness Programs**: Institutions should implement wellness programs that focus on physical and mental health, helping residents balance their demanding schedules with self-care routines.
3. **Code of Conduct**: A clear and accessible code of conduct should outline the expected ethical standards, rules regarding substance abuse, and consequences for violations. This ensures that resident doctors are aware of the importance of maintaining good character.

SUMMARY

Maintaining no addiction and upholding a high standard of character are essential for resident doctors to succeed in their training and professional careers. Addiction can lead to significant personal, professional, and legal consequences, undermining both the doctor's future and the health of their patients. A strong moral character, grounded in ethics, empathy, and professionalism, is foundational to effective healthcare practice. By resisting temptations and maintaining a disciplined and ethical approach, resident doctors can navigate their challenging roles, ensuring personal success and contributing to the betterment of patient care and the healthcare system at large.

CHAPTER 14; MESSAGE FOR MD RESIDENTS AND CONCLUDING REMARKS

Message for MD Residents

As an MD resident, you are at a pivotal stage of your medical career, transitioning from theoretical learning to hands-on clinical practice. The next few years will challenge you in many ways, not just intellectually but emotionally and physically. To succeed, thrive, and make a positive impact in your medical career, keep the following core principles in mind:

Professionalism is Key: The foundation of your medical career lies in maintaining the highest standards of professionalism. This includes being accountable, showing respect to patients and colleagues, adhering to ethical principles, and maintaining a strong moral character. Remember, your actions reflect the values of your institution and the medical profession as a whole.

Avoid Addiction: Addiction, whether to substances like alcohol or drugs or to unhealthy work habits, can severely undermine your ability to provide quality care. The pressures of residency may tempt you, but managing stress, seeking help when needed, and

maintaining a healthy work-life balance will ensure your success and well-being. Recognize the signs of burnout or unhealthy coping mechanisms early and take proactive steps to protect your mental and physical health.

Continual Learning and Self-Reflection: Residency is a time of immense growth. Be committed to lifelong learning, and make self-reflection a regular part of your journey. Every patient interaction, every challenging case, and every mistake is an opportunity to learn and improve. Seek mentorship, ask questions, and never stop evolving as a physician.

Empathy and Compassion: Treat each patient with empathy and respect. Your medical knowledge is critical, but your ability to connect with patients, listen to their concerns, and address their emotional needs will set you apart as a compassionate healer. Remember, medicine is as much about people as it is about science.

Work-Life Balance and Well-being: While residency is demanding, remember that your personal well-being is essential for your success. Maintain balance by dedicating time to self-care, engaging in physical activity, spending time with loved ones, and practicing mindfulness. Healthy doctors provide better care.

Concluding Remarks

The journey through MD residency is one of the most rewarding yet challenging experiences in your medical career. It is a time to develop not just as a clinician but as a compassionate and ethical healthcare professional. The path will test your resilience, intellect, and emotional fortitude, but if you remain grounded in your values and committed to your personal and professional growth, you will emerge as a skilled and compassionate doctor capable of making a meaningful difference in the lives of your patients.

Remember, your future as a doctor is shaped by the choices you make today. Stay focused on your goals, maintain integrity, and always strive for excellence. The dedication and hard work you invest during residency will pave the way for a fulfilling and impactful medical career. Keep your mind and heart open to continuous learning, and never lose sight of why you chose this noble profession in the first place: to serve and heal.

www.ingramcontent.com/pod-product-compliance
Lightning Source LLC
Chambersburg PA
CBHW070358230526
45471CB00006B/2623